Copyright © 2023 by Herman Strange (Author)

All rights reserved. This book or any portion thereof may not be reproduced or used in any manner whatsoever without the express written permission of the publisher except for the use of brief quotations in a book review.

This book is copyright protected. This is only for personal use. You cannot amend, distributor, sell, use, quote or paraphrase any part or the content within this book without the consent of the author. Please note the information contained within this document is for educational and entertainment purposes only. Every attempt has been made to provide accurate, up to date and reliable complete information. No warranties of any kind are expressed or implied.

Readers acknowledge that the author is not engaging in the rendering of legal, financial, medical or professional advice. The content of this book has been derived from various sources. Please consult a licensed professional before attempting any techniques outlined in this book.

By reading this document, the readers agree that under no circumstances are the author responsible for any losses, direct or indirect, which are incurred as a result of the use of information contained within this document, including but not limited to errors, omissions or inaccuracies.

Thank you very much for reading this book.

Title: Managing Stress for Health-Finding Serenity
Subtitle: Techniques for a Happier,
More Relaxed Life

Series: Healthy Habits for Life: Building Sustainable Habits for Optimal Health and Wellness
Author: Serenity Tanner

Table of Contents

Introduction 5
Definition of stress and its effects on physical and mental health 5
The importance of managing stress for overall health and well-being 7

Chapter 1: Understanding Stress 9
The impact of stress on physical and mental health 9
Different types of stress 12
Causes and triggers of stress 15

Chapter 2: Mindfulness and Meditation 18
Benefits of mindfulness and meditation for stress management 18
Different types of meditation techniques 21
Tips for building a daily practice 24

Chapter 3: Yoga and Movement 26
Benefits of yoga and movement for stress management 26
Different types of yoga and movement practices 28
Tips for incorporating movement into daily life 31

Chapter 4: Breathing Techniques 33
Benefits of breathing techniques for stress management 33
Different types of breathing techniques 36
Tips for incorporating breathing into daily life 38

Chapter 5: Cognitive-Behavioral Techniques 40
Benefits of cognitive-behavioral techniques for stress management 40
Different types of cognitive-behavioral techniques 42
Tips for incorporating cognitive-behavioral techniques into daily life 45

Chapter 6: Creating a Stress-Reducing Lifestyle ... 48
Tips for creating a stress-reducing lifestyle 48
The role of sleep, diet, and social connections in stress management 52
Developing a self-care plan for long-term stress management 56

Conclusion 60
Summary of key points 60
Encouragement to take steps towards managing stress for overall health and well-being 63

Potential References 65

Introduction
Definition of stress and its effects on physical and mental health

Stress is a natural part of life and is experienced by everyone at some point. It is a physiological response to a perceived threat or challenge, and can manifest in many different ways, such as feeling anxious, overwhelmed, or irritable. While some level of stress is normal and can even be beneficial in certain situations, chronic or excessive stress can have negative effects on both physical and mental health.

The physiological response to stress involves the release of various hormones, such as adrenaline and cortisol, which prepare the body to respond to the perceived threat or challenge. This response can have a range of effects on the body, including increased heart rate, faster breathing, and increased blood pressure. While this response can be helpful in situations where a quick physical response is needed, such as in a fight-or-flight situation, chronic or excessive stress can lead to long-term damage to the body.

In addition to the physical effects, stress can also have significant effects on mental health. Chronic stress has been linked to increased rates of anxiety, depression, and other mental health conditions. It can also lead to cognitive changes, such as difficulty concentrating, memory problems, and a decreased ability to make decisions.

It is important to note that the effects of stress can vary greatly from person to person. What may be perceived as a stressful situation for one person may not be for another, and the way that stress is experienced and expressed can also differ. However, it is important to recognize the potential negative effects of chronic or excessive stress on both physical and mental health, and to take steps to manage stress in a healthy way.

Throughout this book, we will explore a variety of techniques and strategies for managing stress, including mindfulness and meditation, yoga and movement, breathing techniques, cognitive-behavioral techniques, and lifestyle changes. By learning to manage stress in a healthy way, we can improve our overall health and well-being and live more fulfilling lives.

The importance of managing stress for overall health and well-being

As we discussed earlier, stress is a natural part of life and is experienced by everyone at some point. While some level of stress is normal and can even be beneficial in certain situations, chronic or excessive stress can have negative effects on both physical and mental health. This is why it is important to manage stress in a healthy way.

The negative effects of chronic stress on physical health are well-documented. Long-term stress can lead to a range of health problems, such as high blood pressure, heart disease, and stroke. It can also weaken the immune system, making it more difficult for the body to fight off infections and illnesses. In addition, stress can lead to the development of unhealthy habits, such as overeating, smoking, or excessive drinking, which can further increase the risk of health problems.

In addition to the physical effects, chronic stress can also have significant effects on mental health. It can lead to increased rates of anxiety and depression, and can make it difficult to manage other mental health conditions. Stress can also have a negative impact on relationships, work, and other areas of life, leading to decreased overall satisfaction and well-being.

The good news is that there are a variety of techniques and strategies that can be used to manage stress in a healthy way. By learning to manage stress effectively, we can improve our overall health and well-being. This includes both physical health, such as reducing the risk of health problems, and mental health, such as reducing the risk of mental health conditions and improving overall life satisfaction.

Through the techniques and strategies outlined in this book, we will explore ways to manage stress in a healthy way and improve our overall health and well-being. By taking the time to prioritize our own self-care and manage stress effectively, we can live more fulfilling and enjoyable lives.

Chapter 1: Understanding Stress
The impact of stress on physical and mental health

Stress is an unavoidable part of life, but chronic or excessive stress can have negative effects on both physical and mental health. In this chapter, we will explore how stress impacts physical and mental health and the ways in which chronic stress can contribute to a variety of health problems.

Physical Health

The negative effects of chronic stress on physical health are well-documented. Long-term stress can lead to a range of health problems, such as high blood pressure, heart disease, and stroke. This is because stress triggers the body's "fight or flight" response, which can lead to the release of stress hormones such as adrenaline and cortisol. These hormones can cause an increase in heart rate, blood pressure, and respiration rate, which can be helpful in short-term situations. However, over time, the constant release of stress hormones can lead to a variety of negative health effects.

One of the most significant impacts of chronic stress on physical health is the increased risk of heart disease. The constant release of stress hormones can cause damage to the lining of the blood vessels, leading to inflammation and plaque buildup. This can increase the risk of heart attack and stroke. Chronic stress can also cause an increase in blood pressure, which can lead to hypertension and further increase the risk of heart disease.

Chronic stress can also impact the immune system, making it more difficult for the body to fight off infections and illnesses. This is because the constant release of stress hormones can suppress the immune system, making it less effective. In addition, stress can lead to the development of unhealthy habits, such as overeating, smoking, or excessive drinking, which can further increase the risk of health problems.

Mental Health

In addition to the physical effects, chronic stress can also have significant effects on mental health. It can lead to increased rates of anxiety and depression, and can make it difficult to manage other mental health conditions. Stress can also have a negative impact on relationships, work, and other areas of life, leading to decreased overall satisfaction and well-being.

The relationship between stress and mental health is complex, but it is clear that chronic stress can contribute to the development of mental health problems. This is because stress can cause changes in the brain that can impact mood and behavior. For example, stress can cause a decrease in the production of neurotransmitters such as serotonin and dopamine, which are important for regulating mood.

Chronic stress can also contribute to the development of anxiety and depression. This is because stress can cause a person to feel overwhelmed and unable to cope, leading to feelings of anxiety and helplessness. Over time, this can lead to the development of depression, which is characterized by feelings of sadness, hopelessness, and a loss of interest in activities that were once enjoyable.

In summary, chronic or excessive stress can have negative effects on both physical and mental health. By understanding how stress impacts the body and mind, we can begin to take steps to manage stress effectively and improve our overall health and well-being.

Different types of stress

Stress is a complex phenomenon that can take many different forms. In this chapter, we will explore some of the different types of stress, how they manifest, and the impact they can have on our health and well-being.

Acute Stress

Acute stress is the most common form of stress, and it is usually short-term and caused by a specific event or situation. This type of stress can be positive or negative, and it can be caused by a variety of situations, such as getting a promotion at work, public speaking, or being involved in a minor car accident.

While acute stress is a normal part of life, it can still have negative effects on the body if it is chronic or if it is not effectively managed. For example, chronic acute stress can lead to physical health problems such as headaches, stomach problems, and high blood pressure. It can also contribute to the development of mental health problems such as anxiety and depression.

Episodic Acute Stress

Episodic acute stress is a pattern of stress that occurs when a person experiences acute stress frequently and over an extended period of time. This type of stress is characterized by a sense of being constantly overwhelmed and under pressure, with too many demands and too little time.

People who experience episodic acute stress tend to be highly strung and easily agitated, and they often struggle to manage their emotions and their time effectively. They may feel like they are always running behind, and they may have trouble completing tasks or meeting deadlines.

Chronic Stress

Chronic stress is a long-term form of stress that can be caused by a variety of factors, such as financial problems, job insecurity, or chronic health problems. This type of stress can have serious negative effects on the body, including an increased risk of heart disease, diabetes, and other chronic health problems.

Chronic stress can also have negative effects on mental health, contributing to the development of anxiety, depression, and other mental health problems. People who experience chronic stress may feel hopeless, helpless, and overwhelmed, and they may struggle to maintain healthy relationships, perform well at work, and engage in enjoyable activities.

Traumatic Stress

Traumatic stress is a form of stress that occurs after a person experiences or witnesses a traumatic event, such as a serious accident, natural disaster, or act of violence. This type of stress can have significant negative effects on the body and the mind, and it can lead to the development of post-traumatic stress disorder (PTSD).

PTSD is a mental health condition that is characterized by symptoms such as flashbacks, nightmares, and severe anxiety. People who experience traumatic stress may also struggle with depression, substance abuse, and other mental health problems.

In summary, stress can take many different forms, and each type of stress can have unique effects on the body and the mind. By understanding the different types of stress, we can begin to identify the sources of stress in our lives and take steps to manage stress more effectively.

Causes and triggers of stress

Stress can be caused by a variety of factors, including external circumstances, internal thoughts and beliefs, and physiological responses. In this chapter, we will explore some of the most common causes and triggers of stress, and how they can impact our physical and mental health.

External Stressors

External stressors are factors that are outside of our control, such as environmental factors, social circumstances, and life events. Some common external stressors include:

- Work-related stress: Job-related stress can be caused by factors such as workload, deadlines, interpersonal conflict, and job insecurity.

- Financial stress: Financial stress can be caused by factors such as debt, unemployment, and unexpected expenses.

- Relationship stress: Relationship stress can be caused by factors such as conflict with a partner, family member, or friend, or a lack of social support.

- Environmental stress: Environmental stress can be caused by factors such as noise, pollution, and other physical stressors.

Internal Stressors

Internal stressors are factors that are internal to the individual, such as thoughts, beliefs, and emotions. Some common internal stressors include:

- Negative self-talk: Negative self-talk can include thoughts such as "I'm not good enough," "I can't do this," or "I always mess things up."

- Perfectionism: Perfectionism can lead to stress when a person sets unrealistic expectations for themselves and feels like they must always be perfect.

- Pessimism: Pessimism can lead to stress when a person has a negative outlook on life and sees everything through a negative lens.

- Fear: Fear can be a powerful stressor, and it can be caused by a variety of factors, such as fear of failure, fear of rejection, or fear of the unknown.

Physiological Stressors

Physiological stressors are factors that impact the body and can contribute to the experience of stress. Some common physiological stressors include:

- Lack of sleep: Sleep is critical for physical and mental health, and a lack of sleep can lead to increased stress and anxiety.

- Poor nutrition: A diet that is high in processed foods and low in nutrients can contribute to physical and mental health problems that can increase the experience of stress.

- Lack of exercise: Exercise is an important way to manage stress, and a lack of exercise can contribute to physical and mental health problems that can increase the experience of stress.

In summary, stress can be caused by a variety of factors, including external circumstances, internal thoughts and beliefs, and physiological responses. By understanding the causes and triggers of stress, we can begin to identify the sources of stress in our lives and take steps to manage stress more effectively.

Chapter 2: Mindfulness and Meditation
Benefits of mindfulness and meditation for stress management

Mindfulness and meditation are powerful tools for managing stress and improving overall well-being. Research has shown that these practices can have a wide range of physical and mental health benefits, including reducing stress and anxiety, improving mood, and enhancing cognitive function. In this chapter, we will explore some of the key benefits of mindfulness and meditation for stress management.

Reducing Stress and Anxiety

One of the primary benefits of mindfulness and meditation is their ability to reduce stress and anxiety. When we are stressed or anxious, our bodies activate the "fight or flight" response, which can cause a range of physical and emotional symptoms. Mindfulness and meditation can help to activate the body's relaxation response, which counteracts the stress response and promotes a sense of calm and relaxation.

Improving Mood

Mindfulness and meditation have also been shown to improve mood and emotional well-being. By practicing mindfulness and meditation, we can develop greater awareness of our thoughts and emotions, and learn to respond to them in more positive and constructive ways. This can help to reduce negative emotions such as anger, frustration, and sadness, and promote feelings of joy, gratitude, and contentment.

Enhancing Cognitive Function

In addition to their emotional benefits, mindfulness and meditation can also enhance cognitive function, including attention, memory, and creativity. Research has shown that mindfulness and meditation can help to improve attention and focus, reduce distractibility, and enhance working memory. These cognitive benefits can be particularly helpful for managing stress, as they can help us to stay focused and productive in the face of stressors.

Improving Physical Health

Finally, mindfulness and meditation can also have a range of physical health benefits, including reducing inflammation, improving immune function, and lowering blood pressure. These physical benefits can help to reduce the impact of stress on the body, and promote overall health and well-being.

In summary, mindfulness and meditation are powerful tools for managing stress and improving overall well-being. By reducing stress and anxiety, improving mood and emotional well-being, enhancing cognitive function, and improving physical health, mindfulness and meditation can help us to become more resilient in the face of stressors and better able to cope with the challenges of daily life.

Different types of meditation techniques

Meditation is a powerful tool for managing stress and promoting overall well-being. There are many different types of meditation techniques, each with its own unique benefits and characteristics. In this chapter, we will explore some of the most popular types of meditation techniques, including:

1. Mindfulness Meditation

Mindfulness meditation is a type of meditation that involves bringing your attention to the present moment and noticing your thoughts, feelings, and physical sensations without judgment. This type of meditation can help to reduce stress and anxiety, improve mood and emotional well-being, and enhance cognitive function.

2. Transcendental Meditation

Transcendental meditation is a type of meditation that involves repeating a mantra (a word or phrase) to quiet the mind and achieve a state of deep relaxation. This type of meditation can help to reduce stress and anxiety, improve mood and emotional well-being, and enhance cognitive function.

3. Loving-Kindness Meditation

Loving-kindness meditation is a type of meditation that involves directing positive feelings and intentions towards oneself and others. This type of meditation can help to improve mood and emotional well-being, reduce negative emotions such as anger and frustration, and enhance social connections and relationships.

4. Yoga Meditation

Yoga meditation is a type of meditation that involves combining physical postures (asanas) with meditation and breath work. This type of meditation can help to reduce stress and anxiety, improve mood and emotional well-being, and enhance physical health and fitness.

5. Chakra Meditation

Chakra meditation is a type of meditation that involves focusing on the body's energy centers (chakras) to promote balance and well-being. This type of meditation can help to reduce stress and anxiety, improve mood and emotional well-being, and enhance physical health and vitality.

6. Vipassana Meditation

Vipassana meditation is a type of meditation that involves observing and investigating the body and mind to develop greater awareness and insight. This type of meditation can help to reduce stress and anxiety, improve mood and emotional well-being, and enhance cognitive function.

7. Zen Meditation

Zen meditation is a type of meditation that involves sitting in silence and focusing on the breath or a simple visual object to achieve a state of mental calm and clarity. This type of meditation can help to reduce stress and anxiety, improve mood and emotional well-being, and enhance cognitive function.

In summary, there are many different types of meditation techniques, each with its own unique benefits and characteristics. By exploring different types of meditation, we can find the techniques that work best for our individual needs and preferences, and develop a regular meditation practice to manage stress and promote overall well-being.

Tips for building a daily practice

Building a daily mindfulness and meditation practice is essential to effectively manage stress. Here are some tips to help you get started and establish a regular meditation routine:

1. Start small: It's better to start with a short meditation practice and build up gradually. Try starting with just five or ten minutes per day, and gradually increase the length of your sessions as you become more comfortable.

2. Find a quiet and comfortable space: Choose a quiet and peaceful place where you can sit comfortably and focus on your meditation practice. It can be a room in your home, a garden, or a park. Make sure you won't be disturbed by family members, friends, or pets.

3. Choose a consistent time: Try to meditate at the same time every day to establish a routine. Many people find that meditating first thing in the morning is the most effective way to start the day.

4. Experiment with different techniques: There are many different meditation techniques you can try, including mindfulness meditation, body scan meditation, loving-kindness meditation, and mantra meditation. Experiment with different techniques to find the one that works best for you.

5. Use guided meditations: Guided meditations can be a helpful way to get started and stay focused during your meditation practice. There are many guided meditations available online, including apps like Headspace and Calm.

6. Focus on your breath: One of the simplest and most effective ways to meditate is to focus on your breath. Sit comfortably, close your eyes, and focus on your breath as you inhale and exhale. If your mind starts to wander, gently bring your attention back to your breath.

7. Be patient and persistent: It can take time to establish a regular meditation practice, and it's normal to experience some resistance or difficulty at first. Be patient with yourself and keep trying. Over time, you'll find that meditation becomes easier and more enjoyable.

Remember, building a regular mindfulness and meditation practice takes time and effort, but it can be an incredibly effective way to manage stress and improve your overall well-being. Start small, be consistent, and be kind to yourself as you establish your meditation routine.

Chapter 3: Yoga and Movement
Benefits of yoga and movement for stress management

Yoga and movement practices are widely recognized for their ability to promote relaxation and reduce stress. In this chapter, we will explore the various benefits of yoga and movement for stress management and how these practices can help individuals achieve a greater sense of well-being.

1. Promotes Relaxation Yoga and movement practices encourage relaxation of the body and mind. When we engage in these practices, we focus on our breath, which helps to calm the nervous system and reduce stress.

2. Reduces Muscle Tension Stress often leads to muscle tension, which can cause pain and discomfort. Yoga and movement practices help to reduce muscle tension by stretching and strengthening the muscles. This can lead to greater flexibility and improved posture.

3. Increases Body Awareness Yoga and movement practices increase body awareness. As we move through various poses or exercises, we become more attuned to our bodies and how they feel. This can help us to identify areas of tension and work to release it.

4. Improves Sleep Stress often leads to poor sleep quality. Yoga and movement practices can help to improve

sleep by promoting relaxation and reducing muscle tension. This can lead to a better night's sleep and increased energy levels.

5. Promotes Mindfulness Yoga and movement practices encourage mindfulness, which is the practice of being present in the moment. This can help us to become more aware of our thoughts and feelings and to reduce stress by focusing on the present rather than worrying about the future.

6. Boosts Mood Yoga and movement practices have been shown to improve mood and reduce symptoms of anxiety and depression. This is likely due to the release of endorphins during physical activity and the calming effects of deep breathing and meditation.

7. Increases Social Support Yoga and movement practices can provide a sense of community and social support. By attending classes or practicing with friends, individuals can connect with others who share their interest in reducing stress and improving well-being.

Overall, yoga and movement practices have numerous benefits for stress management and overall health. By incorporating these practices into daily life, individuals can experience greater relaxation, increased body awareness, improved sleep, and a greater sense of well-being.

Different types of yoga and movement practices

Yoga and movement practices have been shown to be effective tools in managing stress and improving overall health and well-being. There are many different types of yoga and movement practices that can be incorporated into a stress management routine, each with its own unique benefits. In this chapter, we will explore some of the most common types of yoga and movement practices that can be used to manage stress.

1. Hatha Yoga Hatha yoga is a gentle form of yoga that is ideal for beginners or those with physical limitations. It focuses on basic poses, breathing techniques, and relaxation, making it an excellent choice for stress relief.

2. Vinyasa Yoga Vinyasa yoga is a more fast-paced form of yoga that focuses on flowing movements and continuous breathing. This type of yoga is great for those who want to build strength and flexibility while also reducing stress.

3. Restorative Yoga Restorative yoga is a gentle, meditative practice that involves holding poses for longer periods of time. It is designed to help the body and mind relax and is a great option for those who are experiencing high levels of stress or anxiety.

4. Yin Yoga Yin yoga is a slow-paced form of yoga that involves holding poses for extended periods of time. It is designed to help improve flexibility and is also an excellent way to reduce stress and improve relaxation.

5. Tai Chi Tai Chi is a form of Chinese martial arts that involves slow, flowing movements and deep breathing. It is a low-impact form of exercise that can be done by people of all ages and fitness levels, making it an excellent choice for stress relief.

6. Pilates Pilates is a form of exercise that focuses on building core strength and improving flexibility. It is a low-impact exercise that can be done by people of all fitness levels and is an excellent way to reduce stress and improve overall well-being.

7. Dance Dancing is a fun and engaging way to reduce stress and improve overall well-being. It can be done in many different forms, from Zumba to ballroom dancing, and is a great way to get moving and reduce tension.

8. Walking Walking is a low-impact form of exercise that can be done by people of all fitness levels. It is an excellent way to reduce stress and improve overall well-being, and can be done almost anywhere.

Incorporating yoga and movement practices into your stress management routine can help you reduce tension, improve relaxation, and improve overall well-being. Whether you prefer a gentle form of yoga or a more vigorous exercise routine, there is a yoga or movement practice that is right for you.

Tips for incorporating movement into daily life

Incorporating movement into your daily routine can be a great way to manage stress and improve your overall health and well-being. Here are some tips for incorporating movement into your daily life:

1. Start small: If you are new to incorporating movement into your routine, start small. You can start with a 10-minute walk in the morning or evening, or try a beginner's yoga video.

2. Find something you enjoy: It's important to find an activity that you enjoy so that you are more likely to stick with it. Whether it's dancing, hiking, swimming, or playing a sport, find an activity that you look forward to doing.

3. Make it a priority: Make movement a priority in your daily routine. Schedule it into your calendar and treat it like any other appointment. When you make movement a priority, you are more likely to stick with it.

4. Take breaks throughout the day: Sitting for long periods of time can be detrimental to your health. Take breaks throughout the day to move your body, whether it's stretching, taking a short walk, or doing a quick yoga flow.

5. Find a workout buddy: Finding a workout buddy can help keep you accountable and make the experience

more enjoyable. You can try new activities together and motivate each other to stay on track.

6. Make it fun: Movement doesn't have to be boring. You can make it fun by trying new activities or incorporating music into your routine. Try a dance class or create a playlist of your favorite songs to listen to while you exercise.

7. Be consistent: Consistency is key when it comes to incorporating movement into your daily routine. Aim to move your body for at least 30 minutes a day, whether it's all at once or broken up into smaller increments throughout the day.

Incorporating movement into your daily routine can have numerous benefits, including reducing stress, improving mood, and boosting overall health and well-being. By following these tips, you can make movement a regular part of your life and reap the benefits that come with it.

Chapter 4: Breathing Techniques
Benefits of breathing techniques for stress management

Breathing techniques are an important tool for managing stress and anxiety. When we feel stressed, our breathing often becomes shallow and rapid, which can worsen our physical and mental symptoms. Practicing breathing techniques can help us to calm our minds and bodies, and promote feelings of relaxation and well-being. In this chapter, we will explore the benefits of breathing techniques for stress management in more detail.

1. Relaxation Response

One of the key benefits of breathing techniques is that they can activate the relaxation response in the body. The relaxation response is the body's natural way of counteracting the stress response. It helps to reduce muscle tension, slow the heart rate, and lower blood pressure. Breathing techniques, such as diaphragmatic breathing, can help to activate the relaxation response, leading to feelings of calm and relaxation.

2. Reduced Anxiety

Breathing techniques can also help to reduce feelings of anxiety. When we feel anxious, our breathing tends to become rapid and shallow, which can exacerbate our symptoms. By practicing breathing techniques, we can slow down our breathing and bring it under our control. This can help to reduce feelings of anxiety and promote a sense of calm.

3. Improved Sleep

Many people struggle with sleep problems due to stress and anxiety. Breathing techniques can be a helpful tool for promoting better sleep. By practicing deep breathing before bed, we can calm our minds and bodies, making it easier to fall asleep and stay asleep throughout the night.

4. Lowered Blood Pressure

High blood pressure is a common side effect of stress. Breathing techniques, such as slow, deep breathing, can help to lower blood pressure and promote better cardiovascular health. By practicing breathing techniques regularly, we can improve our overall health and reduce our risk of developing cardiovascular disease.

5. Increased Focus and Clarity

When we feel stressed, it can be difficult to concentrate and focus on the task at hand. Breathing techniques can help to clear our minds and increase our focus and concentration. By taking a few minutes to practice deep breathing, we can calm our minds and promote a sense of mental clarity.

6. Improved Emotional Well-being

Breathing techniques can also have a positive impact on our emotional well-being. By promoting feelings of relaxation and calm, breathing techniques can help to reduce feelings of depression and anxiety. They can also help us to feel more grounded and centered, which can improve our overall sense of well-being.

In conclusion, breathing techniques are a simple yet effective tool for managing stress and anxiety. They can help to promote feelings of relaxation and well-being, reduce anxiety and depression, and improve our overall health. By incorporating breathing techniques into our daily routine, we can cultivate a sense of calm and resilience, even in the face of stress and adversity.

Different types of breathing techniques

Breathing techniques have long been used as a way to reduce stress and promote relaxation. There are a variety of breathing techniques that can be used for stress management, each with their own unique benefits. In this section, we will explore some of the most common types of breathing techniques and their benefits.

1. Diaphragmatic Breathing: Also known as belly breathing, diaphragmatic breathing involves deep breathing from the diaphragm. This technique involves inhaling deeply through the nose, filling the lungs with air, and exhaling slowly through the mouth. Diaphragmatic breathing is a simple but effective technique that can help reduce stress and promote relaxation.

2. Alternate Nostril Breathing: This breathing technique involves inhaling through one nostril and exhaling through the other, alternating between the two nostrils. This practice has been shown to reduce stress and anxiety, and may also help improve cognitive function and attention.

3. Box Breathing: Box breathing is a simple and effective technique that involves inhaling for a count of four, holding the breath for a count of four, exhaling for a count of four, and holding the breath for a count of four before repeating the cycle. This technique has been shown to reduce

stress and anxiety, and may also help improve sleep and concentration.

4. Equal Breathing: This technique involves inhaling and exhaling for the same length of time, typically for a count of four or six. This technique can help calm the mind and reduce stress and anxiety.

5. Pursed Lip Breathing: This technique involves inhaling deeply through the nose and exhaling slowly through pursed lips, as if blowing out a candle. Pursed lip breathing has been shown to reduce stress and anxiety, and may also help improve lung function.

6. "4-7-8" Breathing: This technique involves inhaling deeply for a count of four, holding the breath for a count of seven, and exhaling slowly for a count of eight. This technique has been shown to reduce stress and anxiety, and may also help improve sleep.

Each of these breathing techniques can be practiced on their own, or combined with other relaxation techniques such as mindfulness and meditation to help manage stress and promote relaxation. Experiment with different techniques to find the ones that work best for you, and try to incorporate them into your daily routine for maximum benefits.

Tips for incorporating breathing into daily life

Learning to manage stress through breathing techniques is a simple and effective way to reduce anxiety and improve overall health and well-being. Incorporating these techniques into your daily routine can help to calm your mind and body, reduce tension, and promote a sense of relaxation. Here are some tips for incorporating breathing techniques into your daily life:

1. Find a quiet space: To fully engage in a breathing practice, it's important to find a quiet space where you won't be disturbed. This could be a designated meditation or yoga space, or simply a comfortable corner of your home where you can sit or lie down without distractions.

2. Make it a habit: Incorporating breathing techniques into your daily routine can be as simple as taking a few deep breaths each morning before you start your day, or doing a quick breathing exercise before bed to help you unwind. Making it a daily habit can help to reinforce the benefits of these techniques and make them a regular part of your self-care routine.

3. Set an intention: Before starting your breathing practice, take a moment to set an intention or focus for your practice. This could be as simple as taking a few deep breaths to help you clear your mind before a busy workday, or using

breathing techniques to help you manage stress and anxiety during a particularly challenging time.

4. Try different techniques: There are many different breathing techniques to choose from, each with its own unique benefits. Experiment with different techniques to find what works best for you, and don't be afraid to mix and match different techniques to create a practice that suits your needs.

5. Focus on the exhale: When practicing breathing techniques, it's important to focus on the exhale as well as the inhale. Exhaling fully can help to release tension and promote relaxation, while also helping to slow down your heart rate and calm your mind.

6. Practice regularly: As with any new habit or skill, consistent practice is key. Try to incorporate breathing techniques into your daily routine, and practice regularly to see the full benefits of these techniques over time.

By incorporating these tips into your daily routine, you can learn to manage stress more effectively and promote a greater sense of relaxation and well-being in your life.

Chapter 5: Cognitive-Behavioral Techniques
Benefits of cognitive-behavioral techniques for stress management

Cognitive-behavioral techniques (CBT) are a type of therapy that focuses on identifying and changing negative thoughts and behaviors that can contribute to stress and anxiety. CBT has been shown to be effective in managing stress and improving mental health. Here are some of the key benefits of CBT for stress management:

1. Provides a structured approach: CBT provides a structured and systematic approach to managing stress, which can be helpful for people who feel overwhelmed or don't know where to start. The therapist works with the client to identify the specific thoughts and behaviors that are contributing to their stress and creates a plan to address them.

2. Targets negative thinking patterns: CBT focuses on identifying and changing negative thinking patterns that can contribute to stress and anxiety. By challenging negative thoughts and replacing them with more realistic and positive ones, clients can learn to reduce their stress levels and improve their overall mental health.

3. Teaches practical coping strategies: CBT teaches clients practical coping strategies that they can use to

manage stress in real-life situations. For example, clients may learn relaxation techniques, problem-solving skills, and effective communication strategies.

4. Helps develop self-awareness: CBT can help clients develop greater self-awareness, which can be useful for identifying triggers and early warning signs of stress. By learning to recognize these signs, clients can take steps to manage their stress before it becomes overwhelming.

5. Is evidence-based: CBT is an evidence-based treatment, which means that it has been rigorously tested and shown to be effective for managing stress and anxiety. There is a wealth of research supporting the use of CBT for a range of mental health issues, including stress and anxiety.

Overall, CBT can be a highly effective approach to managing stress and improving mental health. By providing a structured and practical approach to stress management, CBT can help clients develop the skills and strategies they need to manage stress in their daily lives.

Different types of cognitive-behavioral techniques

Different types of cognitive-behavioral techniques are used in stress management to help individuals identify and modify negative thinking patterns, which can contribute to stress and anxiety. Here are some of the most common techniques used:

1. Cognitive restructuring: This technique involves identifying negative or unhelpful thoughts and replacing them with more positive, realistic ones. The process helps individuals recognize the role of their thoughts in shaping their emotions and behavior, and it can be helpful in reducing stress and anxiety.

2. Problem-solving: Problem-solving is a technique that helps individuals identify and address the root cause of a problem. This approach involves breaking down the problem into smaller parts and developing a plan of action to address each part. By addressing the underlying causes of stress, individuals can reduce their overall stress levels and prevent future stress.

3. Behavioral activation: Behavioral activation is a technique that focuses on increasing positive activities in an individual's life. By increasing the frequency of positive activities, individuals can reduce their overall stress levels and improve their mood. This technique is particularly

helpful for individuals who are struggling with depression or low motivation.

4. Relaxation training: Relaxation techniques, such as deep breathing, progressive muscle relaxation, and visualization, can help individuals reduce their overall stress levels. These techniques help the body relax and reduce tension, which can lead to a reduction in stress and anxiety.

5. Exposure therapy: Exposure therapy is a technique that involves gradually exposing an individual to a feared object or situation. The process helps individuals overcome their fears and reduce their overall stress levels. This technique is particularly helpful for individuals who are struggling with phobias or anxiety disorders.

6. Mindfulness-based stress reduction: Mindfulness-based stress reduction (MBSR) is a technique that involves practicing mindfulness meditation and yoga. The practice helps individuals increase their awareness of the present moment and reduce their overall stress levels. MBSR has been found to be effective in reducing stress, anxiety, and depression.

7. Acceptance and commitment therapy: Acceptance and commitment therapy (ACT) is a technique that focuses on accepting negative thoughts and feelings and committing to values-based actions. The process helps individuals reduce

their overall stress levels by increasing their ability to tolerate uncomfortable thoughts and feelings.

These techniques can be used individually or in combination to help individuals manage their stress levels and improve their overall well-being. It is important to work with a trained mental health professional to determine which techniques will be most effective for your individual needs.

Tips for incorporating cognitive-behavioral techniques into daily life

Cognitive-behavioral techniques are effective tools for managing stress and improving overall mental health. They involve identifying and changing negative thought patterns and behaviors that contribute to stress and anxiety. Cognitive-behavioral techniques can be used in various settings, including therapy sessions and self-help practices. Here are some tips for incorporating cognitive-behavioral techniques into daily life:

1. Practice Mindfulness

Mindfulness is a technique that involves focusing on the present moment without judgment. It can help individuals become more aware of their negative thoughts and feelings and learn to control them. Practicing mindfulness regularly can reduce stress levels and improve overall mental well-being.

2. Identify Triggers

Identifying the triggers that cause stress can help individuals manage their thoughts and behaviors. Once triggers are identified, individuals can work to avoid or manage them. Keeping a journal can help individuals identify their triggers and develop effective strategies for coping with them.

3. Challenge Negative Thoughts

Negative thoughts can lead to increased stress and anxiety. Cognitive-behavioral techniques involve identifying and challenging these negative thoughts. This involves questioning the validity of the negative thought and replacing it with a more positive, rational thought.

4. Set Realistic Goals

Setting realistic goals can help individuals reduce stress and anxiety. Unrealistic goals can lead to feelings of failure and contribute to stress. Setting achievable goals can boost confidence and improve overall well-being.

5. Develop Coping Strategies

Developing effective coping strategies can help individuals manage stress and reduce negative thoughts and behaviors. Coping strategies may include exercise, relaxation techniques, and seeking support from others.

6. Practice Self-Care

Practicing self-care is an essential aspect of cognitive-behavioral techniques. This involves taking care of oneself physically and mentally. Examples of self-care activities include getting enough sleep, eating a healthy diet, and engaging in activities that bring joy and relaxation.

7. Seek Professional Help

While cognitive-behavioral techniques can be effective, individuals may require additional support from a mental health professional. Seeking help from a therapist can provide individuals with the tools they need to manage their stress and improve their overall mental health.

Incorporating cognitive-behavioral techniques into daily life can be challenging, but with practice and persistence, individuals can improve their stress management skills and overall mental well-being.

Chapter 6: Creating a Stress-Reducing Lifestyle
Tips for creating a stress-reducing lifestyle

In the previous chapters, we have discussed various techniques that can be used to manage stress. While these techniques are effective, they are not standalone solutions. Incorporating these techniques into a comprehensive approach to stress management is important to create a stress-reducing lifestyle. In this chapter, we will discuss some tips for creating a stress-reducing lifestyle.

1. Prioritize Self-Care

Self-care is a fundamental aspect of stress management. When you prioritize your physical, emotional, and mental well-being, you're better equipped to handle stress. It's important to make time for activities that you enjoy, such as exercise, reading, or spending time with loved ones. Make sure to prioritize sleep, healthy eating, and staying hydrated as well.

2. Identify and Address Sources of Stress

Understanding the sources of stress in your life is an important step in creating a stress-reducing lifestyle. Take some time to identify the situations, people, or activities that trigger stress in your life. Once you've identified these sources of stress, you can work on creating strategies to address them. This may include learning to say no, setting boundaries, or delegating responsibilities.

3. Practice Mindfulness

Mindfulness is the practice of being present and aware of your thoughts and feelings without judgment. Mindfulness has been shown to be an effective tool for managing stress. Incorporating mindfulness into your daily routine can help you become more aware of your stress triggers, as well as provide an opportunity to relax and recharge. Simple mindfulness practices, such as deep breathing, meditation, or yoga, can be done anywhere and at any time.

4. Stay Organized

Staying organized can help you feel more in control and reduce feelings of stress. Creating a schedule or to-do list can help you prioritize tasks and prevent feeling overwhelmed. Take some time to declutter your physical and digital space as well. When you have an organized space, you're more likely to feel relaxed and less stressed.

5. Connect with Others

Connecting with others can help reduce feelings of stress and promote a sense of well-being. Spend time with friends and family, join a social group or community organization, or volunteer. These activities can help you feel more connected and supported, which is particularly important during times of stress.

6. Practice Gratitude

Gratitude is the practice of focusing on the positive aspects of life. Cultivating a sense of gratitude can help reduce stress and promote feelings of happiness and contentment. Take some time each day to reflect on the things that you're grateful for. This can be as simple as writing down a few things in a gratitude journal, or expressing gratitude to someone in your life.

7. Learn to Relax

Learning to relax is an important aspect of stress management. Relaxation techniques, such as progressive muscle relaxation, deep breathing, or visualization, can help reduce feelings of stress and promote a sense of calm. Incorporating relaxation techniques into your daily routine can help you manage stress more effectively.

8. Take Breaks

Taking breaks is an important aspect of stress management. When you take breaks, you give yourself time to recharge and prevent feeling overwhelmed. Take short breaks throughout the day, such as going for a walk or practicing deep breathing. It's also important to take longer breaks, such as taking a vacation or a day off, to prevent burnout.

In conclusion, creating a stress-reducing lifestyle involves incorporating various techniques into your daily routine. Prioritizing self-care, identifying and addressing sources of stress, practicing mindfulness, staying organized, connecting with others, practicing gratitude, learning to relax, and taking breaks are all important aspects of creating a stress-reducing lifestyle.

The role of sleep, diet, and social connections in stress management

In our fast-paced world, stress has become a common part of our daily lives. While a moderate amount of stress can be beneficial, chronic stress can have adverse effects on our physical and mental health. Therefore, it's important to take steps to manage stress to lead a healthy and fulfilling life. In this chapter, we'll discuss how sleep, diet, and social connections play a crucial role in stress management and how you can incorporate them into your daily life.

The Role of Sleep in Stress Management:

Sleep is an essential component of our health, and it's crucial for stress management. Lack of sleep can have a significant impact on our physical and mental health, leading to increased stress levels. When we're sleep-deprived, our body produces more stress hormones, such as cortisol, which can make us feel more anxious and irritable. Therefore, getting enough sleep is essential for managing stress.

Tips for better sleep:

1. Establish a regular sleep routine: Try to go to bed and wake up at the same time every day, even on the weekends.

2. Create a relaxing sleep environment: Make sure your bedroom is quiet, dark, and cool. Use comfortable pillows and mattresses to ensure a good night's sleep.

3. Limit caffeine and alcohol intake: Avoid drinking caffeinated beverages, such as coffee and tea, in the late afternoon and evening.

4. Turn off electronics: Try to avoid using electronic devices before bedtime, as the blue light emitted by screens can interfere with sleep.

The Role of Diet in Stress Management:

What we eat can also have an impact on our stress levels. Eating a healthy, balanced diet can help us manage stress better. Studies have shown that consuming a diet high in fruits, vegetables, whole grains, and lean protein can help lower stress levels. In contrast, a diet high in sugar, processed foods, and saturated fats can increase stress levels.

Tips for a healthy diet:

1. Eat a variety of foods: Make sure to eat a balanced diet with a variety of fruits, vegetables, whole grains, and lean protein.

2. Limit processed and sugary foods: Try to avoid processed foods, sugary snacks, and sweetened beverages, as they can increase stress levels.

3. Stay hydrated: Drink plenty of water and avoid sugary drinks and caffeine.

The Role of Social Connections in Stress Management:

Social connections play a crucial role in managing stress. Having a support system can help us cope with stressful situations and provide a sense of belonging and emotional support. On the other hand, social isolation can increase stress levels and lead to negative health outcomes.

Tips for building social connections:

1. Connect with others: Join a social group or club, volunteer, or participate in community events to meet new people.

2. Nurture existing relationships: Make time for your friends and family and maintain regular communication.

3. Seek support when needed: Don't hesitate to reach out to your loved ones or a professional if you're struggling with stress.

Conclusion:

Managing stress is essential for maintaining our physical and mental health. Incorporating healthy habits, such as getting enough sleep, eating a balanced diet, and building social connections, can help us better manage stress in our daily lives. By making small changes to our lifestyle, we can create a stress-reducing environment that promotes overall well-being.

Developing a self-care plan for long-term stress management

Stress is a part of life, and it's impossible to eliminate it entirely. However, by developing a self-care plan for long-term stress management, you can learn to cope with stress effectively and minimize its negative impact on your mental and physical health. A self-care plan involves developing healthy habits, taking care of your mind and body, and ensuring that your lifestyle supports your well-being.

In this section, we will discuss how to develop a self-care plan for long-term stress management.

1. Identify Your Stressors

The first step in developing a self-care plan is to identify the things that cause you stress. This could be work-related stress, financial stress, relationship stress, or any other source of stress in your life. Take some time to reflect on the things that make you feel stressed and overwhelmed.

2. Develop Coping Strategies

Once you have identified your stressors, it's time to develop coping strategies. Coping strategies are actions that you can take to reduce your stress levels and manage your stress effectively. Some effective coping strategies include:

- Mindfulness and meditation: Mindfulness and meditation techniques can help you calm your mind and reduce stress levels.

- Exercise: Exercise is a great way to reduce stress and boost your mood.

- Breathing techniques: Breathing techniques can help you calm your mind and reduce stress levels.

- Cognitive-behavioral techniques: Cognitive-behavioral techniques can help you identify and change negative thought patterns that contribute to stress.

3. Make Time for Self-Care Activities

Self-care activities are activities that help you take care of your mind and body. These activities can include anything that makes you feel happy and relaxed, such as reading a book, taking a hot bath, or going for a walk in nature. Make time for self-care activities every day, even if it's just for a few minutes.

4. Practice Good Sleep Hygiene

Getting enough sleep is essential for good mental and physical health. Practice good sleep hygiene by establishing a consistent sleep routine, avoiding caffeine and alcohol before bedtime, and creating a sleep-conducive environment in your bedroom.

5. Eat a Balanced and Nutritious Diet

Eating a balanced and nutritious diet is essential for good mental and physical health. Make sure that you are getting enough fruits, vegetables, whole grains, and lean protein in your diet. Avoid processed foods, sugary drinks, and excessive amounts of caffeine and alcohol.

6. Build Strong Social Connections

Strong social connections are essential for good mental and physical health. Make time for your friends and family, and participate in social activities that make you happy.

7. Set Realistic Goals

Setting realistic goals can help you manage stress effectively. Break larger goals into smaller, more manageable ones, and celebrate your accomplishments along the way.

8. Learn to Say No

Learning to say no is essential for good stress management. Don't be afraid to set boundaries and say no to things that are not essential or that would add unnecessary stress to your life.

In conclusion, developing a self-care plan for long-term stress management involves identifying your stressors, developing coping strategies, making time for self-care activities, practicing good sleep hygiene, eating a balanced and nutritious diet, building strong social connections, setting realistic goals, and learning to say no. By making these lifestyle changes, you can reduce your stress levels and improve your overall well-being. Remember that it's never too late to start taking care of yourself and that small changes can make a big difference.

Conclusion
Summary of key points

The journey of stress management involves understanding the root causes of stress, how it affects us, and learning various techniques to manage it. Through this guide, we have explored different methods for managing stress, including mindfulness and meditation, yoga and movement, breathing techniques, and cognitive-behavioral techniques. We have also discussed the importance of sleep, diet, and social connections in stress management and how to develop a self-care plan for long-term stress management.

In this chapter, we will summarize the key points discussed in the previous chapters to give an overview of how to manage stress effectively.

1. Understanding stress Stress is a natural response to a perceived threat. However, when stress becomes chronic, it can have a significant impact on both physical and mental health. Different types of stress, including acute stress, chronic stress, and traumatic stress, affect people in different ways. Some of the common causes and triggers of stress include work, family, financial problems, and health issues.

2. Mindfulness and meditation Mindfulness and meditation are practices that can help manage stress by increasing awareness of the present moment and reducing

negative thoughts. Various types of meditation, including mindfulness meditation, loving-kindness meditation, and body scan meditation, can be used to manage stress.

3. Yoga and movement Yoga and movement practices, including tai chi, qigong, and dance, can help reduce stress by increasing relaxation and physical activity levels. Practicing yoga and movement can also improve flexibility, strength, and balance.

4. Breathing techniques Breathing techniques can help manage stress by slowing down the breathing rate and reducing anxiety. Different types of breathing techniques, including diaphragmatic breathing, alternate nostril breathing, and box breathing, can be used to manage stress.

5. Cognitive-behavioral techniques Cognitive-behavioral techniques are based on the idea that thoughts, feelings, and behaviors are interconnected. By changing negative thoughts and behaviors, it is possible to reduce stress. Some of the common cognitive-behavioral techniques include cognitive restructuring, exposure therapy, and relaxation training.

6. Creating a stress-reducing lifestyle Sleep, diet, and social connections play a significant role in stress management. Adequate sleep is essential for physical and mental health, and a healthy diet can help improve mood

and energy levels. Social connections can provide emotional support and help reduce stress levels.

7. Developing a self-care plan for long-term stress management Developing a self-care plan can help manage stress in the long term. A self-care plan should include regular physical activity, a healthy diet, adequate sleep, and social connections. Incorporating stress management techniques, including mindfulness, meditation, yoga, and breathing exercises, can also help manage stress.

In conclusion, stress management is an ongoing process that requires awareness, commitment, and practice. By understanding the causes and triggers of stress and learning various techniques to manage it, it is possible to live a healthier and more fulfilling life. It is essential to incorporate stress management techniques into daily life, develop a self-care plan, and seek support from family, friends, or professionals when necessary. By taking a proactive approach to stress management, it is possible to reduce stress levels and improve overall health and well-being.

Encouragement to take steps towards managing stress for overall health and well-being

Stress is an inevitable part of life, and it can have significant impacts on our physical and mental health if not managed properly. The good news is that there are many effective tools and techniques for managing stress and promoting overall health and well-being.

Throughout this guide, we have explored various strategies for stress management, including mindfulness and meditation, yoga and movement, breathing techniques, cognitive-behavioral techniques, and lifestyle changes. While each of these techniques has its own unique benefits, they all share a common goal: to help us better cope with the stressors of daily life and maintain a sense of balance and inner calm.

It's important to note that stress management is not a one-size-fits-all solution. What works for one person may not work for another. It's essential to explore and experiment with different techniques to find what works best for you. Some people may find that a combination of strategies is the most effective way to manage their stress.

As we conclude this guide, we want to encourage you to take steps towards managing your stress for overall health and well-being. Whether it's incorporating mindfulness and meditation into your daily routine, trying a new yoga class, practicing breathing exercises, or making lifestyle changes, know that taking even small steps towards stress management can have a big impact on your life.

Remember, stress is not something that we have to suffer through alone. Seeking support from friends, family, or a mental health professional can help us better navigate the challenges of stress and promote greater well-being. So don't be afraid to ask for help when you need it.

In summary, stress is a part of life, but it doesn't have to control our lives. With the right tools and support, we can learn to manage stress effectively, improve our overall health and well-being, and live more fulfilling lives. So take a deep breath, start exploring different stress management techniques, and be gentle with yourself as you navigate this journey towards greater balance and inner peace.

THE END

Potential References

Introduction:

American Psychological Association. (2021). Stress effects on the body. https://www.apa.org/topics/stress/body

Chapter 1: Understanding Stress

Mayo Clinic. (2021). Chronic stress puts your health at risk. https://www.mayoclinic.org/healthy-lifestyle/stress-management/in-depth/stress/art-20046037

National Institute of Mental Health. (2021). 5 things you should know about stress. https://www.nimh.nih.gov/health/publications/stress/index.shtml

Chapter 2: Mindfulness and Meditation

Davis, D. M., & Hayes, J. A. (2012). What are the benefits of mindfulness? A practice review of psychotherapy-related research. Psychotherapy, 48(2), 198-208.

Khoury, B., Sharma, M., Rush, S. E., & Fournier, C. (2015). Mindfulness-based stress reduction for healthy individuals: A meta-analysis. Journal of psychosomatic research, 78(6), 519-528.

Chapter 3: Yoga and Movement

Chen, K. M., Chen, M. H., Lin, M. H., Fan, J. T., Lin, H. S., & Li, C. H. (2013). Effects of yoga on stress, stress adaption, and heart rate variability among mental health professionals—a randomized controlled trial. Worldviews on Evidence-Based Nursing, 10(1), 44-53.

Sengupta, P. (2012). Health impacts of yoga and pranayama: A state-of-the-art review. International Journal of Preventive Medicine, 3(7), 444-458.

Chapter 4: Breathing Techniques

Jerath, R., Edry, J. W., Barnes, V. A., & Jerath, V. (2006). Physiology of long pranayamic breathing: Neural respiratory elements may provide a mechanism that explains how slow deep breathing shifts the autonomic nervous system. Medical Hypotheses, 67(3), 566-571.

Ma, X., Yue, Z. Q., Gong, Z. Q., Zhang, H., Duan, N. Y., Shi, Y. T., ... Li, Y. F. (2017). The effect of diaphragmatic breathing on attention, negative affect and stress in healthy adults. Frontiers in psychology, 8, 874.

Chapter 5: Cognitive-Behavioral Techniques

Beck, A. T. (1979). Cognitive therapy and the emotional disorders. International Universities Press.

Hofmann, S. G., Asnaani, A., Vonk, I. J., Sawyer, A. T., & Fang, A. (2012). The efficacy of cognitive behavioral therapy: A review of meta-analyses. Cognitive therapy and research, 36(5), 427-440.

Chapter 6: Creating a Stress-Reducing Lifestyle

Centers for Disease Control and Prevention. (2021). Sleep and sleep disorders. https://www.cdc.gov/sleep/index.html

Harvard T.H. Chan School of Public Health. (2021). Diet and mental health. https://www.hsph.harvard.edu/nutritionsource/healthy-eating-plate/diet-and-mental-health/

Conclusion:

Mayo Clinic. (2021). Stress management. https://www.mayoclinic.org/healthy-lifestyle/stress-management/basics/stress-basics/hlv-20049495

National Institute of Mental Health. (2021). 5 things you should know about stress. https://www.nimh.nih.gov/health/publications/stress/index.shtml